This Fitness and Diet Planner Belongs To:

_____

Start Where You Are!

Progress Tracker

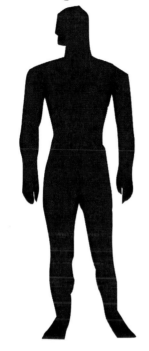

STARTING MEASUREMENTS:

WEIGHT:

LEFT ARM:

RIGHT ARM:

CHEST:

WAIST:

RIGHT THIGH:

LEFT THIGH:

NECK:

My Journey

START DATE:

MY PERSONAL GOALS AND MY "WHY?" :

Progress Tracker

1	2	3	4	5	6	7	8	9	10
11	12	13	14	15	16	17	18	19	20
21	22	23	24	25	26	27	28	29	30
31	32	33	34	35	36	37	38	39	40
41	42	43	44	45	46	47	48	49	50
51	52	53	54	55	56	57	58	59	60
61	62	63	64	65	66	67	68	69	70
71	72	73	74	75	76	77	78	79	80
81	82	83	84	85	86	87	88	89	90

X Your Progress...
It Feels So Good!

30   60   90

My Workout

DATE:

ACTIVITY:	SETS/REPS/DISTANCE/TIME:	CALORIES BURNED? GOAL ACHIEVED?

WATER INTAKE:	SUPPLEMENTS?

Meal Planner

FOOD/TIME/AMOUNT	PROT.	FAT.	CARBS.	CAL.
TOTAL:				

HOW I FELT?/GOALS FOR TOMORROW?   SLEEP:

My Workout

DATE:

ACTIVITY:	SETS/REPS/DISTANCE/TIME:	CALORIES BURNED? GOAL ACHIEVED?

WATER INTAKE:	SUPPLEMENTS?

Meal Planner

FOOD/TIME/AMOUNT	PROT.	FAT.	CARBS.	CAL.
TOTAL:				

HOW I FELT?/GOALS FOR TOMORROW?   SLEEP:

My Workout

DATE:

ACTIVITY:	SETS/REPS/DISTANCE/TIME:	CALORIES BURNED? GOAL ACHIEVED?

WATER INTAKE: ☐ ☐ ☐ ☐ ☐ ☐ ☐	SUPPLEMENTS?

Meal Planner

FOOD/TIME/AMOUNT	PROT.	FAT.	CARDS.	CAL.
TOTAL:				

HOW I FELT?/GOALS FOR TOMORROW?   SLEEP:

My Workout

DATE:

ACTIVITY:	SETS/REPS/DISTANCE/TIME:	CALORIES BURNED? GOAL ACHIEVED?

WATER INTAKE:	SUPPLEMENTS?

Meal Planner

FOOD/TIME/AMOUNT	PROT.	FAT.	CARBS.	CAL.
TOTAL:				

HOW I FELT?/GOALS FOR TOMORROW?   SLEEP:

My Workout

DATE:

ACTIVITY:	SETS/REPS/DISTANCE/TIME:	CALORIES BURNED? GOAL ACHIEVED?

WATER INTAKE:	SUPPLEMENTS?

Meal Planner

FOOD/TIME/AMOUNT	PROT.	FAT.	CARBS.	CAL.
TOTAL:				

HOW I FELT?/GOALS FOR TOMORROW?   SLEEP:

My Workout

DATE:

ACTIVITY:	SETS/REPS/DISTANCE/TIME:	CALORIES BURNED? GOAL ACHIEVED?

WATER INTAKE: ▯ ▯ ▯ ▯ ▯ ▯ ▯ ▯ | SUPPLEMENTS?

Meal Planner

FOOD/TIME/AMOUNT	PROT.	FAT.	CARBS.	CAL.
TOTAL:				

HOW I FELT?/GOALS FOR TOMORROW?   SLEEP:

My Workout

DATE:

ACTIVITY:	SETS/REPS/DISTANCE/TIME:	CALORIES BURNED? GOAL ACHIEVED?

WATER INTAKE:	SUPPLEMENTS?

Meal Planner

FOOD/TIME/AMOUNT	PROT.	FAT.	CARBS.	CAL.
TOTAL:				

HOW I FELT?/GOALS FOR TOMORROW?   SLEEP:

My Workout

ACTIVITY:	SETS/REPS/DISTANCE/TIME:	CALORIES BURNED? GOAL ACHIEVED?

WATER INTAKE:	SUPPLEMENTS?

Meal Planner

FOOD/TIME/AMOUNT	PROT.	FAT.	CARBS.	CAL.
TOTAL:				

HOW I FELT?/GOALS FOR TOMORROW?   SLEEP:

My Workout

DATE:

ACTIVITY:	SETS/REPS/DISTANCE/TIME:	CALORIES BURNED? GOAL ACHIEVED?

WATER INTAKE: ⬜⬜⬜⬜⬜⬜⬜⬜ | SUPPLEMENTS?

Meal Planner

FOOD/TIME/AMOUNT	PROT.	FAT.	CARBS.	CAL.
TOTAL:				

HOW I FELT?/GOALS FOR TOMORROW?   SLEEP:

My Workout

DATE:

ACTIVITY:	SETS/REPS/DISTANCE/TIME:	CALORIES BURNED? GOAL ACHIEVED?

WATER INTAKE:	SUPPLEMENTS?

Meal Planner

FOOD/TIME/AMOUNT	PROT.	FAT.	CARBS.	CAL.
TOTAL:				

HOW I FELT?/GOALS FOR TOMORROW?   SLEEP:

My Workout

DATE:

ACTIVITY:	SETS/REPS/DISTANCE/TIME:	CALORIES BURNED? GOAL ACHIEVED?

WATER INTAKE:	SUPPLEMENTS?

Meal Planner

FOOD/TIME/AMOUNT	PROT.	FAT.	CARBS.	CAL.
TOTAL:				

HOW I FELT?/GOALS FOR TOMORROW?   SLEEP:

My Workout

DATE:

ACTIVITY:	SETS/REPS/DISTANCE/TIME:	CALORIES BURNED? GOAL ACHIEVED?

WATER INTAKE:	SUPPLEMENTS?

Meal Planner

FOOD/TIME/AMOUNT	PROT.	FAT.	CARBS.	CAL.
TOTAL:				

HOW I FELT?/GOALS FOR TOMORROW?   SLEEP:

My Workout

DATE:

ACTIVITY:	SETS/REPS/DISTANCE/TIME:	CALORIES BURNED? GOAL ACHIEVED?

WATER INTAKE: ☐ ☐ ☐ ☐ ☐ ☐ ☐ ☐

SUPPLEMENTS?

Meal Planner

FOOD/TIME/AMOUNT	PROT.	FAT.	CARBS.	CAL.
TOTAL:				

HOW I FELT?/GOALS FOR TOMORROW?   SLEEP:

My Workout

DATE:

ACTIVITY:	SETS/REPS/DISTANCE/TIME:	CALORIES BURNED? GOAL ACHIEVED?

WATER INTAKE: ☐ ☐ ☐ ☐ ☐ ☐ ☐	SUPPLEMENTS?

Meal Planner

FOOD/TIME/AMOUNT	PROT.	FAT.	CARBS.	CAL.
TOTAL:				

HOW I FELT?/GOALS FOR TOMORROW?   SLEEP:

My Workout

DATE:		

ACTIVITY:	SETS/REPS/DISTANCE/TIME:	CALORIES BURNED? GOAL ACHIEVED?

WATER INTAKE:	SUPPLEMENTS?

Meal Planner

FOOD/TIME/AMOUNT	PROT	FAT.	CARBS.	CAL.
TOTAL:				

HOW I FELT?/GOALS FOR TOMORROW?   SLEEP:

My Workout

DATE:

ACTIVITY:	SETS/REPS/DISTANCE/TIME:	CALORIES BURNED? GOAL ACHIEVED?

WATER INTAKE:	SUPPLEMENTS?

Meal Planner

FOOD/TIME/AMOUNT	PROT.	FAT.	CARBS.	CAL.
TOTAL:				

HOW I FELT?/GOALS FOR TOMORROW?   SLEEP:

My Workout

DATE:

ACTIVITY:	SETS/REPS/DISTANCE/TIME:	CALORIES BURNED? GOAL ACHIEVED?

WATER INTAKE:	SUPPLEMENTS?

Meal Planner

FOOD/TIME/AMOUNT	PROT.	FAT	CARBS.	CAL.
TOTAL:				

HOW I FELT?/GOALS FOR TOMORROW?   SLEEP:

My Workout

DATE:

ACTIVITY:	SETS/REPS/DISTANCE/TIME:	CALORIES BURNED? GOAL ACHIEVED?

WATER INTAKE:	SUPPLEMENTS?

Meal Planner

FOOD/TIME/AMOUNT	PROT.	FAT.	CARBS.	CAL.
TOTAL:				

HOW I FELT?/GOALS FOR TOMORROW?   SLEEP:

My Workout

DATE:

ACTIVITY:	SETS/REPS/DISTANCE/TIME:	CALORIES BURNED? GOAL ACHIEVED?

WATER INTAKE: ☐ ☐ ☐ ☐ ☐ ☐ ☐ ☐   SUPPLEMENTS?

Meal Planner

FOOD/TIME/AMOUNT	PROT.	FAT.	CARBS.	CAL.
TOTAL:				

HOW I FELT?/GOALS FOR TOMORROW?   SLEEP:

My Workout

DATE:

ACTIVITY:	SETS/REPS/DISTANCE/TIME:	CALORIES BURNED? GOAL ACHIEVED?

WATER INTAKE: ☐ ☐ ☐ ☐ ☐ ☐ ☐	SUPPLEMENTS?

Meal Planner

FOOD/TIME/AMOUNT	PROT.	FAT.	CARBS.	CAL.
TOTAL:				

HOW I FELT?/GOALS FOR TOMORROW?   SLEEP:

My Workout

DATE:		
ACTIVITY:	**SETS/REPS/DISTANCE/TIME:**	**CALORIES BURNED? GOAL ACHIEVED?**

WATER INTAKE: ☐ ☐ ☐ ☐ ☐ ☐ ☐ ☐ **SUPPLEMENTS?**

Meal Planner

FOOD/TIME/AMOUNT	PROT.	FAT.	CARBS.	CAl
TOTAL:				

HOW I FELT?/GOALS FOR TOMORROW?   **SLEEP:**

My Workout

DATE:

ACTIVITY:	SETS/REPS/DISTANCE/TIME:	CALORIES BURNED? GOAL ACHIEVED?

WATER INTAKE: 🥛 🥛 🥛 🥛 🥛 🥛 🥛 🥛	SUPPLEMENTS?

Meal Planner

FOOD/TIME/AMOUNT	PROT.	FAT.	CARBS.	CAL.
TOTAL:				

HOW I FELT?/GOALS FOR TOMORROW?   SLEEP:

My Workout

DATE:		

ACTIVITY:	SETS/REPS/DISTANCE/TIME:	CALORIES BURNED? GOAL ACHIEVED?

WATER INTAKE:	SUPPLEMENTS?

Meal Planner

FOOD/TIME/AMOUNT	PROT.	FAT.	CARBS.	CAL.
TOTAL:				

HOW I FELT?/GOALS FOR TOMORROW?   SLEEP:

My Workout

DATE:

ACTIVITY:	SETS/REPS/DISTANCE/TIME:	CALORIES BURNED? GOAL ACHIEVED?

WATER INTAKE:	SUPPLEMENTS?

Meal Planner

FOOD/TIME/AMOUNT	PROT.	FAT.	CARBS.	CAL.
TOTAL:				

HOW I FELT?/GOALS FOR TOMORROW?   SLEEP:

My Workout

DATE:

ACTIVITY:	SETS/REPS/DISTANCE/TIME:	CALORIES BURNED? GOAL ACHIEVED?

WATER INTAKE: □ □ □ □ □ □ □ □ □ | SUPPLEMENTS?

Meal Planner

FOOD/TIME/AMOUNT	PROT.	FAT.	CARBS.	CAl
TOTAL:				

HOW I FELT?/GOALS FOR TOMORROW?   SLEEP:

My Workout

DATE:

ACTIVITY:	SETS/REPS/DISTANCE/TIME:	CALORIES BURNED? GOAL ACHIEVED?

WATER INTAKE:	SUPPLEMENTS?

Meal Planner

FOOD/TIME/AMOUNT	PROT.	FAT.	CARBS.	CAL.
TOTAL:				

HOW I FELT?/GOALS FOR TOMORROW?   SLEEP:

My Workout

DATE:

ACTIVITY:	SETS/REPS/DISTANCE/TIME:	CALORIES BURNED? GOAL ACHIEVED?

WATER INTAKE:	SUPPLEMENTS?

Meal Planner

FOOD/TIME/AMOUNT	PROT.	FAT.	CARBS.	CAL.
TOTAL:				

HOW I FELT?/GOALS FOR TOMORROW?   SLEEP:

My Workout

DATE:

ACTIVITY:	SETS/REPS/DISTANCE/TIME:	CALORIES BURNED? GOAL ACHIEVED?

WATER INTAKE:	SUPPLEMENTS?

Meal Planner

FOOD/TIME/AMOUNT	PROT.	FAT.	CARBS.	CAL.
TOTAL:				

HOW I FELT?/GOALS FOR TOMORROW?   SLEEP:

My Workout

DATE:

ACTIVITY:	SETS/REPS/DISTANCE/TIME:	CALORIES BURNED? GOAL ACHIEVED?

WATER INTAKE:	SUPPLEMENTS?

Meal Planner

FOOD/TIME/AMOUNT	PROT.	FAT.	CARBS.	CAL.
TOTAL:				

HOW I FELT?/GOALS FOR TOMORROW?   SLEEP:

My Workout

DATE:

ACTIVITY:	SETS/REPS/DISTANCE/TIME:	CALORIES BURNED? GOAL ACHIEVED?

WATER INTAKE: ☐ ☐ ☐ ☐ ☐ ☐ ☐ ☐	SUPPLEMENTS?

Meal Planner

FOOD/TIME/AMOUNT	PROT.	FAT.	CARBS.	CAL.
TOTAL:				

HOW I FELT?/GOALS FOR TOMORROW?   SLEEP:

Progress Tracker

MEASUREMENTS: **LOSS/GAIN**

WEIGHT:
LEFT ARM:
RIGHT ARM:
CHEST:
WAIST:
RIGHT THIGH:
LEFT THIGH:
NECK:

30 days! YOU MADE IT!

My Journey

HOW WAS THE FIRST 30 DAYS?

GOALS FOR THE NEXT 30 DAYS:

One day at a time…

My Workout

DATE:

ACTIVITY:	SETS/REPS/DISTANCE/TIME:	CALORIES BURNED? GOAL ACHIEVED?

WATER INTAKE: ☐ ☐ ☐ ☐ ☐ ☐ ☐ ☐ | SUPPLEMENTS?

Meal Planner

FOOD/TIME/AMOUNT	PROT.	FAT.	CARBS.	CAL.
TOTAL:				

HOW I FELT?/GOALS FOR TOMORROW?   SLEEP:

My Workout

DATE:

ACTIVITY:	SETS/REPS/DISTANCE/TIME:	CALORIES BURNED? GOAL ACHIEVED?

WATER INTAKE: 🥛 🥛 🥛 🥛 🥛 🥛 🥛 🥛 | SUPPLEMENTS?

Meal Planner

FOOD/TIME/AMOUNT	PROT.	FAT.	CARBS.	CAL.
TOTAL:				

HOW I FELT?/GOALS FOR TOMORROW?   SLEEP:

My Workout

DATE:

ACTIVITY:	SETS/REPS/DISTANCE/TIME:	CALORIES BURNED? GOAL ACHIEVED?

WATER INTAKE:	SUPPLEMENTS?

Meal Planner

FOOD/TIME/AMOUNT	PROT.	FAT.	CARBS.	CAL.
TOTAL:				

HOW I FELT?/GOALS FOR TOMORROW?   SLEEP:

My Workout

DATE:

ACTIVITY:	SETS/REPS/DISTANCE/TIME:	CALORIES BURNED? GOAL ACHIEVED?

WATER INTAKE: ⬜⬜⬜⬜⬜⬜⬜⬜ | SUPPLEMENTS?

Meal Planner

FOOD/TIME/AMOUNT	PROT.	FAT.	CARBS.	CAL.
TOTAL:				

HOW I FELT?/GOALS FOR TOMORROW?   SLEEP:

My Workout

DATE:

ACTIVITY:	SETS/REPS/DISTANCE/TIME:	CALORIES BURNED? GOAL ACHIEVED?

WATER INTAKE:	SUPPLEMENTS?

Meal Planner

FOOD/TIME/AMOUNT	PROT.	FAT.	CARBS.	CAL.
TOTAL:				

HOW I FELT?/GOALS FOR TOMORROW?   SLEEP:

My Workout

DATE:

ACTIVITY:	SETS/REPS/DISTANCE/TIME:	CALORIES BURNED? GOAL ACHIEVED?

WATER INTAKE: | SUPPLEMENTS?

Meal Planner

FOOD/TIME/AMOUNT	PROT.	FAT.	CARBS.	CAL.
TOTAL:				

HOW I FELT?/GOALS FOR TOMORROW?   SLEEP:

My Workout

DATE:

ACTIVITY:	SETS/REPS/DISTANCE/TIME:	CALORIES BURNED? GOAL ACHIEVED?

WATER INTAKE: ☐ ☐ ☐ ☐ ☐ ☐ ☐	SUPPLEMENTS?

Meal Planner

FOOD/TIME/AMOUNT	PROT.	FAT.	CARBS.	CAL.
TOTAL:				

HOW I FELT?/GOALS FOR TOMORROW?   SLEEP:

My Workout

DATE:

ACTIVITY:	SETS/REPS/DISTANCE/TIME:	CALORIES BURNED? GOAL ACHIEVED?

WATER INTAKE: | SUPPLEMENTS?

Meal Planner

FOOD/TIME/AMOUNT	PROT.	FAT.	CARBS.	CAL.
TOTAL:				

HOW I FELT?/GOALS FOR TOMORROW?   SLEEP:

My Workout

DATE:

ACTIVITY:	SETS/REPS/DISTANCE/TIME:	CALORIES BURNED? GOAL ACHIEVED?

WATER INTAKE:	SUPPLEMENTS?

Meal Planner

FOOD/TIME/AMOUNT	PROT.	FAT.	CARBS.	CAL.
TOTAL:				

HOW I FELT?/GOALS FOR TOMORROW?   SLEEP:

My Workout

DATE:

ACTIVITY:	SETS/REPS/DISTANCE/TIME:	CALORIES BURNED? GOAL ACHIEVED?

WATER INTAKE:	SUPPLEMENTS?

Meal Planner

FOOD/TIME/AMOUNT	PROT.	FAT.	CARBS.	CAL
TOTAL:				

HOW I FELT?/GOALS FOR TOMORROW?   SLEEP:

My Workout

DATE:

ACTIVITY:	SETS/REPS/DISTANCE/TIME:	CALORIES BURNED? GOAL ACHIEVED?

WATER INTAKE:	SUPPLEMENTS?

Meal Planner

FOOD/TIME/AMOUNT	PROT.	FAT.	CARBS.	CAL.
TOTAL:				

HOW I FELT?/GOALS FOR TOMORROW?   SLEEP:

My Workout

DATE:

ACTIVITY:	SETS/REPS/DISTANCE/TIME:	CALORIES BURNED? GOAL ACHIEVED?

WATER INTAKE: SUPPLEMENTS?

Meal Planner

FOOD/TIME/AMOUNT	PROT.	FAT.	CARBS.	CAL.
TOTAL:				

HOW I FELT?/GOALS FOR TOMORROW?   SLEEP:

My Workout

DATE:

ACTIVITY:	SETS/REPS/DISTANCE/TIME:	CALORIES BURNED? GOAL ACHIEVED?

WATER INTAKE:	SUPPLEMENTS?

Meal Planner

FOOD/TIME/AMOUNT	PROT.	FAT.	CARBS.	CAL.
TOTAL:				

HOW I FELT?/GOALS FOR TOMORROW?   SLEEP:

My Workout

DATE:

ACTIVITY:	SETS/REPS/DISTANCE/TIME:	CALORIES BURNED? GOAL ACHIEVED?

WATER INTAKE: □ □ □ □ □ □ □ □ | **SUPPLEMENTS?**

Meal Planner

FOOD/TIME/AMOUNT	PROT.	FAT.	CARBS.	CAL.
TOTAL:				

HOW I FELT?/GOALS FOR TOMORROW?   SLEEP:

My Workout

DATE:

ACTIVITY:	SETS/REPS/DISTANCE/TIME:	CALORIES BURNED? GOAL ACHIEVED?

WATER INTAKE:	SUPPLEMENTS?

Meal Planner

FOOD/TIME/AMOUNT	PROT.	FAT.	CARBS.	CAL.
TOTAL:				

HOW I FELT?/GOALS FOR TOMORROW?   SLEEP:

My Workout

DATE:

ACTIVITY:	SETS/REPS/DISTANCE/TIME:	CALORIES BURNED? GOAL ACHIEVED?

WATER INTAKE:	SUPPLEMENTS?

Meal Planner

FOOD/TIME/AMOUNT	PROT.	FAT.	CARBS.	CAL.
TOTAL:				

HOW I FELT?/GOALS FOR TOMORROW?   SLEEP:

My Workout

DATE:

ACTIVITY:	SETS/REPS/DISTANCE/TIME:	CALORIES BURNED? GOAL ACHIEVED?

WATER INTAKE:	SUPPLEMENTS?

Meal Planner

FOOD/TIME/AMOUNT	PROT.	FAT.	CARBS.	CAL.
TOTAL:				

HOW I FELT?/GOALS FOR TOMORROW?   SLEEP:

My Workout

DATE:

ACTIVITY:	SETS/REPS/DISTANCE/TIME:	CALORIES BURNED? GOAL ACHIEVED?

WATER INTAKE:	SUPPLEMENTS?

Meal Planner

FOOD/TIME/AMOUNT	PROT.	FAT.	CARBS.	CAL.
TOTAL:				

HOW I FELT?/GOALS FOR TOMORROW?   SLEEP:

My Workout

DATE:

ACTIVITY:	SETS/REPS/DISTANCE/TIME:	CALORIES BURNED? GOAL ACHIEVED?

WATER INTAKE: ☐ ☐ ☐ ☐ ☐ ☐ ☐ ☐	SUPPLEMENTS?

Meal Planner

FOOD/TIME/AMOUNT	PROT.	FAT.	CARBS.	CAL.
TOTAL:				

HOW I FELT?/GOALS FOR TOMORROW?   SLEEP:

My Workout

DATE:

ACTIVITY:	SETS/REPS/DISTANCE/TIME:	CALORIES BURNED? GOAL ACHIEVED?

WATER INTAKE:	SUPPLEMENTS?

Meal Planner

FOOD/TIME/AMOUNT	PROT.	FAT.	CARBS.	CAL.
TOTAL:				

HOW I FELT?/GOALS FOR TOMORROW?   SLEEP:

My Workout

DATE:

ACTIVITY:	SETS/REPS/DISTANCE/TIME:	CALORIES BURNED? GOAL ACHIEVED?

WATER INTAKE: ☐ ☐ ☐ ☐ ☐ ☐ ☐ ☐	SUPPLEMENTS?

Meal Planner

FOOD/TIME/AMOUNT	PROT.	FAT.	CARBS.	CAL.
TOTAL:				

HOW I FELT?/GOALS FOR TOMORROW?   SLEEP:

My Workout

DATE:

ACTIVITY:	SETS/REPS/DISTANCE/TIME:	CALORIES BURNED? GOAL ACHIEVED?

WATER INTAKE:	SUPPLEMENTS?

Meal Planner

FOOD/TIME/AMOUNT	PROT.	FAT.	CARBS.	CAL.
TOTAL:				

HOW I FELT?/GOALS FOR TOMORROW?   SLEEP:

My Workout

DATE:

ACTIVITY:	SETS/REPS/DISTANCE/TIME:	CALORIES BURNED? GOAL ACHIEVED?

WATER INTAKE: ☐ ☐ ☐ ☐ ☐ ☐ ☐ ☐   SUPPLEMENTS?

Meal Planner

FOOD/TIME/AMOUNT	PROT.	FAT.	CARBS.	CAL.
TOTAL:				

HOW I FELT?/GOALS FOR TOMORROW?   SLEEP:

My Workout

	DATE:	

ACTIVITY:	SETS/REPS/DISTANCE/TIME:	CALORIES BURNED? GOAL ACHIEVED?

WATER INTAKE:	SUPPLEMENTS?

Meal Planner

FOOD/TIME/AMOUNT	PROT.	FAT.	CARBS.	CAL.
TOTAL:				

HOW I FELT?/GOALS FOR TOMORROW?   SLEEP:

My Workout

DATE:

ACTIVITY:	SETS/REPS/DISTANCE/TIME:	CALORIES BURNED? GOAL ACHIEVED?

WATER INTAKE: ☐ ☐ ☐ ☐ ☐ ☐ ☐ ☐ | **SUPPLEMENTS?**

Meal Planner

FOOD/TIME/AMOUNT	PROT.	FAT.	CARBS.	CAL.
TOTAL:				

HOW I FELT?/GOALS FOR TOMORROW?   SLEEP:

My Workout

DATE:

ACTIVITY:	SETS/REPS/DISTANCE/TIME:	CALORIES BURNED? GOAL ACHIEVED?

WATER INTAKE:	SUPPLEMENTS?

Meal Planner

FOOD/TIME/AMOUNT	PROT.	FAT.	CARBS.	CAL.
TOTAL:				

HOW I FELT?/GOALS FOR TOMORROW?   SLEEP:

My Workout

DATE:

ACTIVITY:	SETS/REPS/DISTANCE/TIME:	CALORIES BURNED? GOAL ACHIEVED?

WATER INTAKE: ▯ ▯ ▯ ▯ ▯ ▯ ▯	SUPPLEMENTS?

Meal Planner

FOOD/TIME/AMOUNT	PROT.	FAT.	CARBS.	CAL.
TOTAL:				

HOW I FELT?/GOALS FOR TOMORROW?   SLEEP:

My Workout

DATE:

ACTIVITY:	SETS/REPS/DISTANCE/TIME:	CALORIES BURNED? GOAL ACHIEVED?

WATER INTAKE:	SUPPLEMENTS?

Meal Planner

FOOD/TIME/AMOUNT	PROT.	FAT.	CARBS.	CAI
TOTAL:				

HOW I FELT?/GOALS FOR TOMORROW?   SLEEP:

My Workout

DATE:

ACTIVITY:	SETS/REPS/DISTANCE/TIME:	CALORIES BURNED? GOAL ACHIEVED?

WATER INTAKE: ▯ ▯ ▯ ▯ ▯ ▯ ▯ ▯	SUPPLEMENTS?

Meal Planner

FOOD/TIME/AMOUNT	PROT.	FAT.	CARBS.	CAL.
TOTAL:				

HOW I FELT?/GOALS FOR TOMORROW?   SLEEP:

My Workout

DATE:		

ACTIVITY:	SETS/REPS/DISTANCE/TIME:	CALORIES BURNED? GOAL ACHIEVED?

WATER INTAKE:	SUPPLEMENTS?

Meal Planner

FOOD/TIME/AMOUNT	PROT.	FAT.	CARBS.	CAL.
TOTAL:				

HOW I FELT?/GOALS FOR TOMORROW?   SLEEP:

Progress Tracker

MEASUREMENTS: **LOSS/GAIN**

| WEIGHT: |
| RIGHT ARM: |
| LEFT ARM: |
| CHEST: |
| WAIST: |
| RIGHT THIGH: |
| LEFT THIGH: |
| NECK: |

60 Days! YOU MADE IT!

☆

My Journey

HOW WAS THE PREVIOUS 30 DAYS?

GOALS FOR THE NEXT 30 DAYS:

One day at a time...

My Workout

DATE:

ACTIVITY:	SETS/REPS/DISTANCE/TIME:	CALORIES BURNED? GOAL ACHIEVED?

WATER INTAKE:	SUPPLEMENTS?

Meal Planner

FOOD/TIME/AMOUNT	PROT.	FAT.	CARBS.	CAL.
TOTAL:				

HOW I FELT?/GOALS FOR TOMORROW?   SLEEP:

My Workout

DATE:

ACTIVITY:	SETS/REPS/DISTANCE/TIME:	CALORIES BURNED? GOAL ACHIEVED?

WATER INTAKE: □ □ □ □ □ □ □ | SUPPLEMENTS?

Meal Planner

FOOD/TIME/AMOUNT	PROT.	FAT.	CARBS.	CAL.
TOTAL:				

HOW I FELT?/GOALS FOR TOMORROW?   SLEEP:

My Workout

DATE:

ACTIVITY:	SETS/REPS/DISTANCE/TIME:	CALORIES BURNED? GOAL ACHIEVED?

WATER INTAKE: ☐ ☐ ☐ ☐ ☐ ☐ ☐ ☐	SUPPLEMENTS?

Meal Planner

FOOD/TIME/AMOUNT	PROT.	FAT.	CARBS.	CAL.
TOTAL:				

HOW I FELT?/GOALS FOR TOMORROW?   SLEEP:

My Workout

DATE:

ACTIVITY:	SETS/REPS/DISTANCE/TIME:	CALORIES BURNED? GOAL ACHIEVED?

WATER INTAKE:	SUPPLEMENTS?

Meal Planner

FOOD/TIME/AMOUNT	PROT.	FAT.	CARBS.	CAL.
TOTAL:				

HOW I FELT?/GOALS FOR TOMORROW?   SLEEP:

My Workout

DATE:

ACTIVITY:	SETS/REPS/DISTANCE/TIME:	CALORIES BURNED? GOAL ACHIEVED?

WATER INTAKE:	SUPPLEMENTS?

Meal Planner

FOOD/TIME/AMOUNT	PROT.	FAT.	CARBS.	CAL.
TOTAL:				

HOW I FELT?/GOALS FOR TOMORROW?   SLEEP:

My Workout

DATE:

ACTIVITY:	SETS/REPS/DISTANCE/TIME:	CALORIES BURNED? GOAL ACHIEVED?

WATER INTAKE: ⬜ ⬜ ⬜ ⬜ ⬜ ⬜ ⬜ ⬜	SUPPLEMENTS?

Meal Planner

FOOD/TIME/AMOUNT	PROT.	FAT.	CARBS.	CAL.
TOTAL:				

HOW I FELT?/GOALS FOR TOMORROW?   SLEEP:

My Workout

DATE:

ACTIVITY:	SETS/REPS/DISTANCE/TIME:	CALORIES BURNED? GOAL ACHIEVED?

WATER INTAKE: ☐ ☐ ☐ ☐ ☐ ☐ ☐	SUPPLEMENTS?

Meal Planner

FOOD/TIME/AMOUNT	PROT.	FAT.	CARBS.	CAL.
TOTAL:				

HOW I FELT?/GOALS FOR TOMORROW?   SLEEP:

My Workout

DATE:

ACTIVITY:	SETS/REPS/DISTANCE/TIME:	CALORIES BURNED? GOAL ACHIEVED?

WATER INTAKE:	SUPPLEMENTS?

Meal Planner

FOOD/TIME/AMOUNT	PROT.	FAT.	CARBS.	CAL.
TOTAL:				

HOW I FELT?/GOALS FOR TOMORROW?   SLEEP:

My Workout

DATE:

ACTIVITY:	SETS/REPS/DISTANCE/TIME:	CALORIES BURNED? GOAL ACHIEVED?

WATER INTAKE:	SUPPLEMENTS?

Meal Planner

FOOD/TIME/AMOUNT	PROT.	FAT.	CARBS.	CAL.
TOTAL:				

HOW I FELT?/GOALS FOR TOMORROW?   SLEEP:

My Workout

DATE:

ACTIVITY:	SETS/REPS/DISTANCE/TIME:	CALORIES BURNED? GOAL ACHIEVED?

WATER INTAKE: ☐ ☐ ☐ ☐ ☐ ☐ ☐ ☐ | SUPPLEMENTS?

Meal Planner

FOOD/TIME/AMOUNT	PROT.	FAT.	CARBS.	CAL.
TOTAL:				

HOW I FELT?/GOALS FOR TOMORROW?　　　　　　SLEEP:

My Workout

DATE:

ACTIVITY:	SETS/REPS/DISTANCE/TIME:	CALORIES BURNED? GOAL ACHIEVED?

WATER INTAKE: SUPPLEMENTS?

Meal Planner

FOOD/TIME/AMOUNT	PROT.	FAT.	CARBS.	CAL.
TOTAL:				

HOW I FELT?/GOALS FOR TOMORROW?   SLEEP:

My Workout

DATE:

ACTIVITY:	SETS/REPS/DISTANCE/TIME:	CALORIES BURNED? GOAL ACHIEVED?

WATER INTAKE: ▯ ▯ ▯ ▯ ▯ ▯ ▯ ▯   SUPPLEMENTS?

Meal Planner

FOOD/TIME/AMOUNT	PROT.	FAT.	CARBS.	CAL.
TOTAL:				

HOW I FELT?/GOALS FOR TOMORROW?   SLEEP:

My Workout

DATE:

ACTIVITY:	SETS/REPS/DISTANCE/TIME:	CALORIES BURNED? GOAL ACHIEVED?

WATER INTAKE: ☐ ☐ ☐ ☐ ☐ ☐ ☐ ☐	SUPPLEMENTS?

Meal Planner

FOOD/TIME/AMOUNT	PROT.	FAT.	CARBS.	CAL.
TOTAL:				

HOW I FELT?/GOALS FOR TOMORROW?   SLEEP:

My Workout

DATE:

ACTIVITY:	SETS/REPS/DISTANCE/TIME:	CALORIES BURNED? GOAL ACHIEVED?

WATER INTAKE:	SUPPLEMENTS?

Meal Planner

FOOD/TIME/AMOUNT	PROT.	FAT.	CARBS.	CAL.
TOTAL:				

HOW I FELT?/GOALS FOR TOMORROW?   SLEEP:

My Workout

DATE:

ACTIVITY:	SETS/REPS/DISTANCE/TIME:	CALORIES BURNED? GOAL ACHIEVED?

WATER INTAKE:	SUPPLEMENTS?

Meal Planner

FOOD/TIME/AMOUNT	PROT.	FAT.	CARBS.	CAL.
TOTAL:				

HOW I FELT?/GOALS FOR TOMORROW?   SLEEP:

My Workout

DATE:

ACTIVITY:	SETS/REPS/DISTANCE/TIME:	CALORIES BURNED? GOAL ACHIEVED?

WATER INTAKE: | SUPPLEMENTS?

Meal Planner

FOOD/TIME/AMOUNT	PROT.	FAT.	CARBS.	CAL.
TOTAL:				

HOW I FELT?/GOALS FOR TOMORROW?   SLEEP:

My Workout

DATE:

ACTIVITY:	SETS/REPS/DISTANCE/TIME:	CALORIES BURNED? GOAL ACHIEVED?

WATER INTAKE:	SUPPLEMENTS?

Meal Planner

FOOD/TIME/AMOUNT	PROT.	FAT.	CARBS.	CAL.
TOTAL:				

HOW I FELT?/GOALS FOR TOMORROW?   SLEEP:

My Workout

ACTIVITY:	SETS/REPS/DISTANCE/TIME:	CALORIES BURNED? GOAL ACHIEVED?

WATER INTAKE:	SUPPLEMENTS?

Meal Planner

FOOD/TIME/AMOUNT	PROT.	FAT.	CARBS.	CAL.
TOTAL:				

HOW I FELT?/GOALS FOR TOMORROW?   SLEEP:

My Workout

DATE:

ACTIVITY:	SETS/REPS/DISTANCE/TIME:	CALORIES BURNED? GOAL ACHIEVED?

WATER INTAKE: ☐ ☐ ☐ ☐ ☐ ☐ ☐	SUPPLEMENTS?

Meal Planner

FOOD/TIME/AMOUNT	PROT.	FAT.	CARBS.	CAL.
TOTAL:				

HOW I FELT?/GOALS FOR TOMORROW?   SLEEP:

My Workout

DATE:

ACTIVITY:	SETS/REPS/DISTANCE/TIME:	CALORIES BURNED? GOAL ACHIEVED?

WATER INTAKE: ▢ ▢ ▢ ▢ ▢ ▢ ▢ ▢   SUPPLEMENTS?

Meal Planner

FOOD/TIME/AMOUNT	PROT.	FAT.	CARBS.	CAL.
TOTAL:				

HOW I FELT?/GOALS FOR TOMORROW?   SLEEP:

My Workout

DATE:

ACTIVITY:	SETS/REPS/DISTANCE/TIME:	CALORIES BURNED? GOAL ACHIEVED?

WATER INTAKE:	SUPPLEMENTS?

Meal Planner

FOOD/TIME/AMOUNT	PROT.	FAT.	CARBS.	CAL.
TOTAL:				

HOW I FELT?/GOALS FOR TOMORROW?   SLEEP:

My Workout

DATE:

ACTIVITY:	SETS/REPS/DISTANCE/TIME:	CALORIES BURNED? GOAL ACHIEVED?

WATER INTAKE: ▯ ▯ ▯ ▯ ▯ ▯ ▯ ▯	SUPPLEMENTS?

Meal Planner

FOOD/TIME/AMOUNT	PROT.	FAT.	CARBS.	CAL.
TOTAL:				

HOW I FELT?/GOALS FOR TOMORROW?   SLEEP:

My Workout

DATE:

ACTIVITY:	SETS/REPS/DISTANCE/TIME:	CALORIES BURNED? GOAL ACHIEVED?

WATER INTAKE:	SUPPLEMENTS?

Meal Planner

FOOD/TIME/AMOUNT	PROT.	FAT.	CARBS.	CAL.
TOTAL:				

HOW I FELT?/GOALS FOR TOMORROW?   SLEEP:

My Workout

DATE:

ACTIVITY:	SETS/REPS/DISTANCE/TIME:	CALORIES BURNED? GOAL ACHIEVED?

WATER INTAKE:	SUPPLEMENTS?

Meal Planner

FOOD/TIME/AMOUNT	PROT.	FAT.	CARBS.	CAL.
TOTAL:				

HOW I FELT?/GOALS FOR TOMORROW?   SLEEP:

My Workout

DATE:

ACTIVITY:	SETS/REPS/DISTANCE/TIME:	CALORIES BURNED? GOAL ACHIEVED?

WATER INTAKE:	SUPPLEMENTS?

Meal Planner

FOOD/TIME/AMOUNT	PROT.	FAT.	CARBS.	CAL.
TOTAL:				

HOW I FELT?/GOALS FOR TOMORROW?   SLEEP:

My Workout

DATE:

ACTIVITY:	SETS/REPS/DISTANCE/TIME:	CALORIES BURNED? GOAL ACHIEVED?

WATER INTAKE: ☐ ☐ ☐ ☐ ☐ ☐ ☐ ☐	SUPPLEMENTS?

Meal Planner

FOOD/TIME/AMOUNT	PROT.	FAT.	CARBS.	CAL.
TOTAL:				

HOW I FELT?/GOALS FOR TOMORROW?   SLEEP:

My Workout

DATE:

ACTIVITY:	SETS/REPS/DISTANCE/TIME:	CALORIES BURNED? GOAL ACHIEVED?

WATER INTAKE:	SUPPLEMENTS?

Meal Planner

FOOD/TIME/AMOUNT	PROT.	FAT.	CARBS.	CAL.
TOTAL:				

HOW I FELT?/GOALS FOR TOMORROW?   SLEEP:

My Workout

DATE:

ACTIVITY:	SETS/REPS/DISTANCE/TIME:	CALORIES BURNED? GOAL ACHIEVED?

WATER INTAKE: ☐ ☐ ☐ ☐ ☐ ☐ ☐	SUPPLEMENTS?

Meal Planner

FOOD/TIME/AMOUNT	PROT.	FAT.	CARBS.	CAL.
TOTAL:				

HOW I FELT?/GOALS FOR TOMORROW?   SLEEP:

My Workout

DATE:

ACTIVITY:	SETS/REPS/DISTANCE/TIME:	CALORIES BURNED? GOAL ACHIEVED?

WATER INTAKE:	SUPPLEMENTS?

Meal Planner

FOOD/TIME/AMOUNT	PROT.	FAT.	CARBS.	CAL.
TOTAL:				

HOW I FELT?/GOALS FOR TOMORROW?   SLEEP:

My Workout

DATE:

ACTIVITY:	SETS/REPS/DISTANCE/TIME:	CALORIES BURNED? GOAL ACHIEVED?

WATER INTAKE: ▯ ▯ ▯ ▯ ▯ ▯ ▯ ▯ | SUPPLEMENTS?

Meal Planner

FOOD/TIME/AMOUNT	PROT.	FAT.	CARBS.	CAL.
TOTAL:				

HOW I FELT?/GOALS FOR TOMORROW?   SLEEP:

Progress Tracker

MEASUREMENTS: LOSS/GAIN

WEIGHT:
LEFT ARM:
RIGHT ARM:
CHEST:
WAIST:
RIGHT THIGH:
LEFT THIGH:
NECK:

90 Days! YOU MADE IT!

My Journey

HOW WAS THE PREVIOUS 30 DAYS?

GOALS FOR YOUR NEXT 30 DAYS:

One day at a time...

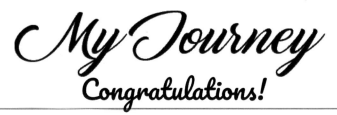

My Journey

Congratulations!

CURRENT WEIGHT/FITNESS LEVEL VS PREVIOUS:

HOW DO YOU FEEL ABOUT THE PROGRESS YOU'VE MADE?

GOALS FOR YOUR NEXT 90 DAYS:

WRITE 5 POSITIVE THINGS ABOUT YOUR BODY:

Believe. Achieve. Succeed!

Notes

One day at a time...

Remember to keep tracking your fitness and diet to stay accountable. Every little step you take helps you to see how far you've come and make progress.

For your next 90 day planner please take a look at some of our other fun cover designs listed under our author name :

"Good Life Publishing"

Stay Motivated and Happy Tracking!

Made in United States
North Haven, CT
07 March 2022

16891159R00057